Hope and Healing: Nourishing Recipes cookbook for Cancer Patients

By Eric A. Sherman

Tables of contents

Chapter 1.introduction to the purpose of cancer cookbook

Chapter 2: Breakfast and Brunch Recipes

Chapter 3: Lunch and Dinner Recipes

Chapter 4: Snacks and Appetizers

Chapter 5: Desserts and Treats

Chapter 6: Tips for Meal Planning and Preparation

Chapter 1.introduction to the purpose of cancer cookbook

The purpose of the cancer cookbook is to provide cancer patients and their families with a collection of nutritious and delicious recipes that can support their health and wellbeing during treatment. Cancer treatment can be physically and emotionally challenging, and proper nutrition is essential to maintain strength, energy, and overall health. This cookbook aims to make mealtime enjoyable and stress-free by providing easy-to-follow recipes that incorporate cancer-fighting ingredients and are gentle on the stomach. By promoting healthy eating habits, the cookbook can help improve the quality of life for cancer patients and their families

Overview of the types of foods that can help support cancer patients during treatment

Cancer treatments such as chemotherapy, radiation therapy, and surgery can have significant effects on the body, including nausea, vomiting, fatigue, loss of appetite, and weakened immune system. Eating a healthy diet during cancer treatment is essential to support the body's needs for nutrients, maintain a healthy weight, and promote overall well-being.

Here are some types of foods that can help support cancer patients during treatment:

Fruits and vegetables: Eating a variety of colorful fruits and vegetables can help provide essential vitamins, minerals, and antioxidants to support the immune system and help protect against cellular damage. Aim for at least 5 servings per day.

Lean protein sources: Foods like poultry, fish, eggs, beans, and lentils can help support muscle mass and aid in tissue repair.

Whole grains: Eating whole grains like brown rice, quinoa, and whole-wheat bread can help provide fiber, which can help with digestion and bowel regularity.

Healthy fats: Incorporating healthy fats like olive oil, avocado, nuts, and seeds can help provide essential fatty acids, which can help reduce inflammation and support brain health.

Fluids: Drinking plenty of water and other fluids like herbal tea, low-fat milk, and vegetable juices can help prevent dehydration and aid in digestion.

It is also essential to avoid or limit certain foods that can be detrimental to health, such as processed foods, high-fat foods, and sugary drinks.

Additionally, cancer patients may benefit from working with a registered dietitian who can provide personalized recommendations and support during treatment.

Explanation of how certain nutrients and compounds in these foods can help boost immunity, reduce inflammation, and improve overall health.

Certainly! There are many nutrients and compounds found in certain foods that can help boost immunity, reduce inflammation, and improve overall health. Here are some examples:

Vitamin C: Found in citrus fruits, berries, kiwi, and many other fruits and vegetables, vitamin C is a powerful antioxidant that can help boost the immune system and reduce inflammation.

Zinc: Found in nuts, seeds, seafood, and whole grains, zinc is an essential mineral that helps support immune function and reduce inflammation.

Omega-3 fatty acids: Found in fatty fish, such as salmon and sardines, as well as flaxseeds and chia seeds, omega-3 fatty acids have anti-inflammatory properties and can help reduce the risk of chronic diseases.

Probiotics: Found in fermented foods, such as yogurt, kefir, and kimchi, probiotics are beneficial bacteria that can help improve gut health and support immune function.

Polyphenols: Found in fruits, vegetables, tea, and dark chocolate, polyphenols are antioxidants that can help reduce inflammation and improve overall health.

Vitamin D: Found in fatty fish, egg yolks, and fortified foods, vitamin D is essential for immune function and can help reduce inflammation.

Fiber: Found in whole grains, fruits, and vegetables, fiber helps support gut health and can help reduce inflammation.

By incorporating these nutrient-rich foods into your diet, you can help boost your immune system, reduce inflammation, and improve your overall health.

Healthy Meal Suggestions.

Without knowing which specific foods you are referring to, here are some general suggestions for incorporating a variety of healthy foods into meals and snacks throughout the day:

Start the day with a healthy breakfast that includes whole grains, protein, and healthy fats. Some options include oatmeal with nuts and fruit, a veggie omelette, or a smoothie with spinach, berries, and almond milk.

For snacks, try to choose foods that are high in fiber and protein, such as fruits with nut butter, Greek yogurt with berries, or a handful of nuts.
Make sure to include plenty of vegetables with your meals. You can add them to omelettes, salads, stir-fries, soups, or roast them as a side dish.
Incorporate whole grains into your meals, such as brown rice, quinoa, or whole wheat pasta.

For protein, try to choose lean options like chicken, fish, tofu, or legumes.

Add healthy fats to your meals by including foods like avocado, nuts, seeds, or olive oil.

Stay hydrated throughout the day by drinking plenty of water, and try to limit sugary drinks like soda or juice.

Remember, a balanced and varied diet is key for optimal health, so try to mix up your meals and snacks as much as possible.

Chapter 2: Breakfast and Brunch Recipes

Nutritious Breakfast Recipes:
A selection of nutritious and easy-to-prepare breakfast and brunch recipes

Sure! Here are some ideas for nutritious and easy-to-prepare breakfast and brunch recipes:

Avocado Toast: Toast a slice of whole grain bread and top with mashed avocado, a sprinkle of salt and pepper, and any other toppings you like, such as sliced tomatoes, a poached egg, or crumbled feta cheese.

Greek Yogurt Parfait: Layer Greek yogurt, fresh berries, and granola in a glass or jar for a healthy and filling breakfast.

Smoothie Bowl: Blend frozen fruit, milk or yogurt, and a handful of greens like spinach or kale to create a thick and creamy smoothie. Pour into a bowl and top with sliced fruit, granola, and nuts.

Banana Pancakes: Mash a ripe banana and whisk in an egg and a tablespoon of flour. Cook like regular pancakes on a non-stick pan and top with your favorite toppings, such as nut butter, honey, or sliced fruit.

Scrambled Eggs with Veggies: Whisk together eggs and a splash of milk, then cook in a non-stick pan with chopped veggies like bell peppers, onions, and spinach. Serve with whole grain toast.

Breakfast Burrito: Scramble eggs with black beans, bell peppers, and cheese. Wrap in a whole grain tortilla and serve with salsa and avocado.
Overnight Oats: Combine rolled oats, milk, Greek yogurt, and your choice of sweetener in a jar and let sit overnight. In the morning, top with fresh fruit and nuts.

Egg Muffin Cups: Whisk together eggs, cheese, and chopped veggies, then pour into a greased muffin tin and bake until set. Serve with whole grain toast. Chia Seed Pudding: Mix chia seeds, milk, and sweetener in a jar and let sit in the fridge overnight. In the morning, top with sliced fruit and nuts.

Smoked Salmon and Cream Cheese Toast: Toast a slice of whole grain bread and spread with cream cheese. Top with smoked salmon, sliced red onion, and capers.

These are just a few ideas to get you started. Enjoy!

Emphasis on foods that are gentle on the stomach and easy to digest, as well as those that provide sustained energy throughout the morning.

If you're looking for foods that are gentle on the stomach and easy to digest while also providing sustained energy throughout the morning, here are some suggestions:

Oatmeal: Oatmeal is a great choice for a gentle, easy-to-digest breakfast that will keep you feeling full and energized. It's high in fiber, which helps regulate digestion, and it's also a complex carbohydrate that releases energy slowly over time.

Greek yogurt: Greek yogurt is an excellent source of protein, which can help you feel full and satisfied throughout the morning. It's also low in lactose, making it easier on the stomach for those who are sensitive to dairy.

Bananas: Bananas are rich in fiber, potassium, and other nutrients that help regulate digestion and provide sustained energy. They're also easy to digest and gentle on the stomach.

Toast with nut butter: Whole-grain toast with almond or peanut butter is an excellent source of complex carbohydrates and protein, providing sustained energy while also being easy to digest.

Smoothies: Smoothies made with low-fiber fruits like bananas, berries, and melons can be a great way to get a nutrient-packed breakfast that's easy on the stomach. Adding protein powder or Greek yogurt can also help keep you feeling full and satisfied.

Eggs: Eggs are a great source of protein and healthy fats, which can help keep you feeling full and energized throughout the morning. Scrambled or boiled eggs are easy to digest and gentle on the stomach.

Remember to pay attention to your body's individual needs and preferences when choosing foods that are gentle on the stomach and easy to digest. If you have specific dietary restrictions or sensitivities, be sure to choose foods that meet your needs.

Chapter 3: Lunch and Dinner Recipes

Delicious Nutritious Recipes

A variety of recipes for main dishes, sides, and salads that are both delicious and nutritious

Sure, here are some recipes for main dishes, sides, and salads that are both delicious and nutritious:

Main Dishes:

Grilled Chicken with Mango Salsa: Marinate chicken breasts in a mixture of lime juice, honey, and chili powder, then grill until cooked through. Serve with a homemade salsa made with diced mango, red onion, jalapeño, lime juice, and cilantro.

Quinoa and Vegetable Stir-Fry: Cook quinoa according to package instructions, then stir-fry with your favorite vegetables such as bell peppers, broccoli, carrots, and snow peas. Add a sauce made with soy sauce, rice vinegar, ginger, garlic, and honey.

Baked Salmon with Roasted Vegetables: Season salmon fillets with salt, pepper, and garlic powder, then bake in the oven. Serve with roasted vegetables such as asparagus, zucchini, and cherry tomatoes.

Sides:

Roasted Sweet Potato Wedges: Cut sweet potatoes into wedges, toss with olive oil, salt, and smoked paprika, and roast in the oven until crispy and tender.

Sauteed Garlic Spinach: Heat olive oil in a pan, add minced garlic and spinach, and sauté until wilted. Season with salt, pepper, and a squeeze of lemon juice.

Grilled Zucchini with Lemon and Parmesan: Slice zucchini lengthwise, brush with olive oil, and grill until tender. Top with grated Parmesan cheese and a squeeze of lemon juice.
Salads:

Kale and Quinoa Salad: Massage kale leaves with olive oil, lemon juice, and salt to tenderize them. Mix with cooked quinoa, cherry tomatoes, cucumber, avocado, and a honey mustard dressing.
Grilled Peach and Arugula Salad: Grill sliced peaches until caramelized, then toss with arugula, goat cheese, toasted almonds, and a balsamic vinaigrette.
Greek Salad with Chickpeas: Mix chopped romaine lettuce, diced cucumber, cherry tomatoes, Kalamata olives, feta cheese, and chickpeas. Dress with a Greek vinaigrette made with red wine vinegar, olive oil, oregano, and garlic.
Enjoy!

Healthy diet for cancer.

Emphasis on using fresh, whole ingredients and incorporating a variety of cancer-fighting foods

A diet that emphasizes fresh, whole ingredients and incorporates a variety of cancer-fighting foods can play a crucial role in reducing the risk of cancer and promoting overall health. Here are some key principles to keep in mind:

Focus on fresh, whole foods: Eating a diet rich in fresh fruits and vegetables, whole grains, and lean protein sources like fish and poultry can provide essential nutrients and fiber to support a healthy immune system and reduce the risk of cancer.

Incorporate cancer-fighting foods: Some foods have been shown to have specific cancer-fighting properties. These include cruciferous vegetables like broccoli and cauliflower, berries like blueberries and raspberries, green tea, turmeric, garlic, and mushrooms. Incorporating these foods into your diet can provide a range of health benefits.

Choose healthy fats: Fats are an essential part of a healthy diet, but it's important to choose the right kinds. Unsaturated fats found in sources like nuts, seeds, and olive oil can help reduce inflammation and support heart health, while saturated and trans fats found in processed and fried foods can increase the risk of cancer.

Limit processed and red meat: Processed meats like bacon, sausage, and deli meats have been linked to an increased risk of cancer. Red meat should also be consumed in moderation, as it has been associated with a   health. Avoid sugary drinks and limit alcohol consumption, which can increase the risk of certain cancers.

By following these principles and making healthy food choices a priority, you can help reduce your risk of cancer and support your overall health and well-being.

Chapter 4: Snacks and Appetizers

Healthy Snacks Suggestions.

Suggestions for healthy, satisfying snacks and appetizers that can be enjoyed throughout the day.

Sure, here are some suggestions for healthy, satisfying snacks and appetizers that you can enjoy throughout the day:

Fresh Fruit: Cut up some fresh fruit, like apples, bananas, berries, or oranges, and enjoy as a snack.

Vegetable Crudites: Cut up some carrots, celery, bell peppers, and cucumbers and serve with hummus, guacamole, or salsa.

Yogurt Parfait: Layer Greek yogurt, granola, and fresh fruit for a protein-packed snack.

Nuts and Seeds: Snack on a handful of almonds, cashews, pumpkin seeds, or sunflower seeds for a satisfying crunch.

Roasted Chickpeas: Toss chickpeas with olive oil, salt, and your favorite spices and roast in the oven for a crunchy snack.

Rice Cakes: Top rice cakes with almond butter, avocado, or hummus for a satisfying snack.

Hard-Boiled Eggs: Boil a batch of eggs and keep them in the fridge for a quick and easy snack.

Air-Popped Popcorn: Pop some popcorn in an air popper and season with salt, pepper, or nutritional yeast for a healthy snack.

Edamame: Boil or steam edamame and sprinkle with salt for a protein-packed snack.

Veggie Chips: Slice sweet potatoes, beets, or kale thinly and bake in the oven for crispy veggie chips.

Remember to listen to your body and eat when you're hungry, and stop when you're full.
Energizing Digestion Ingredients.
Emphasis on using ingredients that provide sustained energy and help combat nausea and other digestive issues.

When it comes to choosing ingredients for sustained energy and to combat nausea and other digestive issues, here are a few suggestions:

Complex carbohydrates: Complex carbohydrates like whole grains, legumes, and starchy vegetables are digested slowly, providing a steady supply of energy. These foods also contain fiber, which helps regulate digestion and prevent nausea. Good options include brown rice, quinoa, lentils, sweet potatoes, and whole-grain bread.

Lean proteins: Protein is important for maintaining energy levels and helping to build and repair tissues. Lean sources of protein like chicken, turkey, fish, tofu, and beans are easier on the digestive system than high-fat or heavily processed meats.

Healthy fats: While fats are often associated with indigestion, healthy fats like those found in nuts, seeds, and avocados can help regulate digestion and provide sustained energy. These foods are also rich in nutrients like vitamin E, which can help reduce inflammation in the digestive tract.

Ginger: Ginger is a natural anti-inflammatory and has been shown to help alleviate nausea and vomiting. Try adding fresh ginger to tea, smoothies, or stir-fries, or sipping on ginger tea throughout the day.

Peppermint: Peppermint has a calming effect on the digestive system and can help alleviate symptoms of nausea and indigestion. Sip on peppermint tea or add fresh peppermint leaves to water or smoothies.

Hydration: Dehydration can cause fatigue and contribute to digestive issues. Make sure to drink plenty of water throughout the day, and consider sipping on hydrating beverages like coconut water or electrolyte-enhanced sports drinks if you're engaging in strenuous activity.

Healthy snack recipe ideas.
Recipes could include homemade granola bars, dips made with beans or avocado, roasted nuts, and fresh fruit and vegetable plates.

Great suggestions! Here are some recipes to try:

Homemade Granola Bars:

Ingredients:

2 cups old-fashioned rolled oats
1/2 cup chopped nuts (almonds, pecans, or walnuts)
1/2 cup honey
1/4 cup coconut oil
1/4 cup brown sugar
1/2 teaspoon salt
1/2 teaspoon cinnamon
1/2 cup dried fruit (raisins, cranberries, or chopped apricots)
Instructions:

Preheat oven to 350°F (175°C).
Spread oats and nuts on a baking sheet and bake for 10-15 minutes, until lightly toasted.
In a small saucepan, combine honey, coconut oil, brown sugar, salt, and cinnamon. Cook over

medium heat, stirring occasionally, until mixture comes to a boil.

In a large mixing bowl, combine toasted oats and nuts with dried fruit. Pour hot honey mixture over the oat mixture and stir well.

Press mixture firmly into an 8x8 inch baking pan that has been lined with parchment paper.

Bake for 20-25 minutes, until golden brown.

Let cool for 10 minutes, then cut into bars. Allow to cool completely before storing in an airtight container.

Bean Dip:

Ingredients:

1 can (15 ounces) black beans, drained and rinsed
1/2 cup salsa
1/2 cup shredded cheddar cheese
1/4 cup chopped fresh cilantro
Juice of 1 lime
Salt and pepper to taste

Instructions:

In a food processor or blender, combine beans, salsa, cheese, cilantro, and lime juice. Puree until smooth.
Season with salt and pepper to taste.
Serve with tortilla chips or cut-up vegetables.
Avocado Dip:

Ingredients:

2 ripe avocados
Juice of 1 lime
1/4 cup chopped fresh cilantro
1/4 teaspoon ground cumin
Salt and pepper to taste
Instructions:

Cut avocados in half, remove pit, and scoop out flesh into a medium bowl.

Add lime juice, cilantro, cumin, salt, and pepper. Mash with a fork until desired consistency is reached.

Serve with tortilla chips or cut-up vegetables.

Roasted Nuts:

Ingredients:

2 cups mixed nuts (almonds, cashews, and/or pecans)

2 tablespoons melted butter

1 tablespoon honey

1 teaspoon ground cinnamon

1/4 teaspoon salt

Instructions:

Preheat oven to 350°F (175°C).

In a large bowl, combine nuts, melted butter, honey, cinnamon, and salt. Toss to coat.

Spread nut mixture out in a single layer on a baking sheet.

Bake for 10-15 minutes, stirring occasionally, until nuts are lightly browned and fragrant.

Let cool completely before storing in an airtight container.

Fresh Fruit and Vegetable Plate:

Ingredients:

Assorted fresh fruits (strawberries, blueberries, grapes, pineapple, etc.)

Assorted fresh vegetables (carrots, cucumbers, cherry tomatoes, etc.)

Hummus or ranch dressing for dipping

Instructions:

Wash and prepare fruits and vegetables.

Arrange on a large platter or individual plates.

Serve with hummus or ranch dressing for dipping.

Chapter 5: Desserts and Treats

Nutritious Dessert Ideas.

Ideas for desserts and treats that are both tasty and nutritious

Here are some ideas for desserts and treats that are both tasty and nutritious:

Fruit salad: A mixture of fresh fruits can be a delicious and nutritious dessert. You can mix fruits like apples, bananas, berries, mangoes, and pineapples.

Greek yogurt with berries: Greek yogurt is high in protein, and it can be topped with fresh berries for a sweet and nutritious treat.

Baked apples: Baked apples can be a healthy dessert that's also satisfying. Simply core the apples, fill them with raisins, cinnamon, and a little bit of honey, and bake them until they're tender.

Dark chocolate-covered almonds: Dark chocolate is rich in antioxidants, and almonds are a great source of protein and healthy fats. Combine the two for a delicious and nutritious snack.

Peanut butter banana bites: Cut a banana into slices, spread a little peanut butter on each slice, and top with chopped nuts or shredded coconut.

Chia seed pudding: Chia seeds are a great source of fiber and protein, and they can be used to make a creamy and delicious pudding. Mix chia seeds with almond milk and sweetener of your choice and let it set in the fridge.

Homemade energy bars: You can make energy bars at home using healthy ingredients like oats, nuts, seeds, and dried fruits.

Frozen yogurt popsicles: Mix together Greek yogurt, honey, and fresh fruit like berries, pour it into popsicle molds, and freeze for a healthy and refreshing treat.

Fruit sorbet: Blend frozen fruit with a little bit of honey or agave syrup and serve for a refreshing and nutritious dessert.

Sweet potato brownies: Swap out regular flour for sweet potato flour, and use dark chocolate for a rich and healthier version of brownies.

Natural Sweeteners and Cancer-Fighting Foods.

Emphasis on using natural sweeteners and incorporating cancer-fighting ingredients like berries, dark chocolate, and nuts.

Using natural sweeteners like honey, maple syrup, and dates is a great way to add sweetness to your diet without relying on highly processed sugars. These natural sweeteners not only provide a delicious flavor, but they also have a lower glycemic index, which means they are absorbed more slowly and can help regulate blood sugar levels.

Incorporating cancer-fighting ingredients like berries, dark chocolate, and nuts can also be beneficial for your health. Berries are rich in antioxidants, which can help protect cells from damage and reduce the risk of cancer. Dark chocolate contains flavonoids, which have been shown to have anti-cancer properties. Nuts are a great source of healthy fats and also contain antioxidants and other compounds that may help protect against cancer.

When it comes to incorporating these ingredients into your diet, there are many delicious and healthy options. For example, you could add berries to your morning oatmeal, sprinkle nuts on top of a salad, or enjoy a small piece of dark chocolate as a dessert. By making small changes to your diet and incorporating these cancer-fighting ingredients, you can help support your overall health and wellbeing.

Healthy Recipe Ideas.

Recipes could include smoothie bowls, fruit sorbets, baked goods made with whole grains and natural sweeteners, and healthy versions of classic desserts like chocolate mousse and cheesecake.

Here are some recipes for the items you mentioned:

Smoothie Bowl Recipe:

Ingredients:

1 cup frozen mixed berries

1 frozen banana

1/2 cup almond milk

1/4 cup Greek yogurt

1 tbsp honey

1 tbsp chia seeds

1/4 cup granola

Sliced fruit for topping

Instructions:

Combine frozen berries, frozen banana, almond milk, Greek yogurt, honey, and chia seeds in a blender and blend until smooth.

Pour smoothie into a bowl and top with granola and sliced fruit.

Fruit Sorbet Recipe:

Ingredients:

4 cups frozen mixed berries

1/4 cup honey

1/4 cup lemon juice

Instructions:

Combine frozen berries, honey, and lemon juice in a blender or food processor and blend until smooth.
Pour mixture into a loaf pan and freeze for 4-6 hours, stirring occasionally.
Scoop sorbet into bowls and serve.
Whole Grain Chocolate Chip Cookies Recipe:

Ingredients:

1 cup whole wheat flour
1/2 tsp baking soda
1/2 tsp salt
1/2 cup coconut oil, melted
1/2 cup honey
1 egg
1 tsp vanilla extract
1/2 cup dark chocolate chips
Instructions:

Preheat oven to 350°F and line a baking sheet with parchment paper.

In a medium bowl, whisk together whole wheat flour, baking soda, and salt.

In a separate bowl, mix together melted coconut oil, honey, egg, and vanilla extract.

Add dry ingredients to wet ingredients and mix until combined.

Fold in dark chocolate chips.

Drop dough by rounded tablespoons onto prepared baking sheet and bake for 10-12 minutes or until golden brown.

Allow cookies to cool on the baking sheet for a few minutes before transferring to a wire rack to cool completely.

Healthy Chocolate Mousse Recipe:

Ingredients:

1 avocado

1/4 cup cocoa powder

1/4 cup honey

1 tsp vanilla extract

Pinch of salt

1/4 cup almond milk

Instructions:

Cut avocado in half and remove the pit.

Scoop the avocado flesh into a blender or food processor.

Add cocoa powder, honey, vanilla extract, salt, and almond milk to the blender and blend until smooth.

Transfer mixture to a bowl or individual ramekins and refrigerate for at least 30 minutes.

Serve chilled.

Healthy Cheesecake Recipe:

Ingredients:

2 cups low-fat Greek yogurt

2 tbsp honey

1 tsp vanilla extract

1/4 cup almond flour

1/4 cup oats

1/4 cup chopped almonds

2 tbsp coconut oil, melted

2 tbsp honey

1/2 tsp cinnamon

Instructions:

Preheat oven to 350°F and line a 9-inch springform pan with parchment paper.

In a medium bowl, mix together Greek yogurt, honey, and vanilla extract.

In a separate bowl, mix together almond flour, oats, chopped almonds, melted coconut oil, honey, and cinnamon.

Press the almond flour mixture into the bottom of the prepared springform pan.

Pour the Greek yogurt mixture over the crust and smooth out the top.

Bake for 30-35 minutes or until the edges are golden brown and the center is set.

Allow cheesecake to cool to room temperature before refrigerating for at least

Chapter 6: Tips for Meal Planning and Preparation

Meal Planning Made Easy.

Suggestions for planning and preparing meals in advance to make the process easier and less stressful

Planning and preparing meals in advance can definitely make the process of cooking easier and less stressful. Here are some suggestions:

Create a meal plan: Before the week begins, take some time to plan out what meals you want to prepare for the week. This will help you to stay organized and ensure that you have all the necessary ingredients on hand.

Make a grocery list: Once you have your meal plan, make a list of all the ingredients you'll need for each recipe. This will help you to avoid last-minute trips to the grocery store.

Prep ingredients ahead of time: Chop vegetables, marinate meats, and make sauces ahead of time so that you can easily put together meals during the week.

Cook in bulk: When you do have time to cook, make extra so that you can freeze leftovers for later meals. This is especially helpful for soups, stews, and casseroles.

Invest in good storage containers: Having good quality containers to store your prepared meals in will make it easier to keep track of what you have on hand and will help you to avoid food waste.

Use a slow cooker or pressure cooker: These appliances can be a real time-saver. You can set them up in the morning before work and come home to a delicious meal that's ready to eat.

Have a backup plan: Sometimes things don't go according to plan, so it's a good idea to have some easy backup meals on hand, like frozen pizzas or pre-made salads.

Remember, the key to successful meal planning and preparation is to find a routine that works for you and to be flexible when things don't go as planned. With a little bit of effort, you can make mealtime less stressful and more enjoyable.

Leftover Storage Tips.

Tips for storing and reheating leftovers to ensure maximum freshness and flavor.

Storing and reheating leftovers properly can help maintain their freshness and flavor. Here are some tips:

Store leftovers in airtight containers: Use containers with tight-fitting lids to keep air out and prevent moisture from escaping.

Label and date leftovers: Write the date on the container so you know when the food was stored. This will help you keep track of how long the food has been stored and when it needs to be used or thrown away.

Refrigerate leftovers promptly: Store leftovers in the refrigerator within two hours after cooking. This will prevent bacteria from growing and keep the food safe to eat.

Store leftovers in the right place: Place leftovers in the coldest part of your refrigerator, which is usually the back or bottom shelf. Avoid storing leftovers in the refrigerator door, as the temperature there can vary.

Reheat leftovers properly: Reheat leftovers to a temperature of at least 165°F (74°C) to kill any bacteria that may have grown. Use a food thermometer to check the temperature.

Use the right reheating method: Some foods are best reheated in the oven, while others are best reheated on the stove or in the microwave. Use the appropriate method for the type of food you are reheating.

Add moisture: Add a bit of moisture to dry leftovers to help them retain their moisture when reheated. This can be done by adding a splash of water, broth, or sauce before reheating.

Reheat in small portions: Reheat small portions of leftovers at a time to ensure even heating and to prevent overcooking.

Don't reheat leftovers more than once: Reheating leftovers more than once can increase the risk of foodborne illness. Only reheat leftovers once and consume them within 3-4 days of being stored.

Adapting recipes to dietary needs.

Advice on how to adapt recipes to fit individual dietary needs and preferences

Adapting recipes to fit individual dietary needs and preferences can seem like a daunting task, but with a few simple tips and tricks, it can be a fun and easy process. Here are some guidelines to help you get started:

Understand the dietary restrictions: The first step in adapting a recipe is to understand the dietary restrictions or preferences of the person you are cooking for. This may include restrictions on certain ingredients, such as dairy or gluten, or preferences for certain types of foods, such as vegetarian or vegan.

Substitute ingredients: Once you understand the dietary restrictions, you can start to substitute ingredients in the recipe to fit those needs. For example, if a recipe calls for milk, you could substitute it with a non-dairy milk like almond or soy milk. If a recipe calls for wheat flour, you could substitute it with a gluten-free flour like rice or oat flour.

Adjust measurements: When substituting ingredients, it's important to adjust the measurements accordingly. For example, if a recipe calls for 1 cup of milk, but you are substituting with almond milk, you may need to adjust the amount to ¾ or ⅔ cups depending on the recipe.

Experiment with spices and seasonings: If a recipe calls for an ingredient that cannot be substituted, like meat, you can experiment with spices and seasonings to add flavor and depth to the dish. For example, you could use a blend of spices like smoked paprika, cumin, and coriander to create a smoky flavor in a vegetarian chili.

Use online resources: There are many online resources available that offer recipes and tips for adapting recipes to fit dietary needs and preferences. These can be a great starting point when you are first learning to adapt recipes.

Remember, adapting recipes takes practice and experimentation. Don't be afraid to try new things and make mistakes. With time and experience, you will become more comfortable and confident in adapting recipes to fit individual dietary needs and preferences.

Healthy Diet and Cancer.

Summary of the benefits of a healthy, cancer-fighting diet.

A healthy, cancer-fighting diet can offer several benefits, including:

Reducing the risk of cancer: Eating a diet that is high in fruits, vegetables, whole grains, and lean protein can help reduce the risk of cancer. These foods are rich in antioxidants, fiber, and other nutrients that can protect against cancer.

Boosting the immune system: Eating a diet that is high in nutrients can help boost the immune system. This can help the body fight off cancer and other diseases.

Lowering inflammation: A diet that is high in processed foods, red meat, and saturated fats can cause inflammation in the body. Chronic inflammation has been linked to the development of cancer, so eating a diet that is low in these foods can help reduce the risk.

Maintaining a healthy weight: Obesity has been linked to several types of cancer. Eating a healthy diet and maintaining a healthy weight can help reduce the risk.

Improving overall health: Eating a healthy diet can also help reduce the risk of other chronic diseases, such as heart disease and diabetes. This can improve overall health and well-being.

Overall, a healthy, cancer-fighting diet should be rich in fruits, vegetables, whole grains, lean protein, and healthy fats. It should also be low in processed foods, red meat, and saturated fats.

Experimenting with Cookbook Recipes.

Encouragement for readers to experiment with the recipes in the cookbook and find what works best for them and their families.

If you're a cookbook enthusiast, you know that one of the most exciting aspects of cooking is experimenting with new recipes. While it can be tempting to stick to the instructions exactly as they're written, it's important to remember that everyone's taste buds are different, and what works for one family might not work for another.

So, don't be afraid to tweak recipes to suit your preferences and dietary needs. If you're not a fan of spicy food, for example, you can reduce the amount of chili powder or omit it altogether. Or, if you're looking to make a recipe healthier, you can try substituting ingredients like butter for olive oil or using whole wheat flour instead of white flour.

It's also important to keep in mind that cooking is a learning process, and you're not always going to get it right the first time. Don't be discouraged if a recipe doesn't turn out the way you expected – take note of what worked and what didn't, and make adjustments for next time.

So, get creative in the kitchen and have fun experimenting with the recipes in your cookbook. Who knows, you might even discover a new family favorite!

Nutrition and Self-Care.

Final thoughts on the importance of nutrition and self-care during cancer treatment.

Nutrition and self-care are essential components of cancer treatment. A cancer diagnosis can be emotionally and physically taxing, and proper nutrition and self-care can help patients maintain their strength and cope with the side effects of cancer treatment.

During cancer treatment, the body's nutritional needs may change, and patients may need to make adjustments to their diet to ensure they are getting the nutrients they need. For example, some cancer treatments can cause nausea, vomiting, and diarrhea, which can make it difficult for patients to eat and absorb nutrients. In such cases, working with a registered dietitian can help patients identify foods that are easy to digest and provide the nutrients they need.

Self-care is equally important during cancer treatment. Cancer patients may experience a range of emotional and physical symptoms, including anxiety, depression, pain, and fatigue. Self-care activities such as exercise, meditation, and relaxation techniques can help patients manage these symptoms and improve their quality of life. Engaging in activities that bring joy and provide a sense of purpose can also help patients maintain a positive outlook and cope with the challenges of cancer treatment.

In conclusion, nutrition and self-care are critical aspects of cancer treatment. Patients should work with their healthcare team to develop a personalized nutrition plan that meets their individual needs and engage in self-care activities that promote physical and emotional well-being. By taking care of themselves, cancer patients can improve their treatment outcomes, reduce side effects, and enhance their overall quality of life.